THE
BIBLE
CURE ®
FOR

CHRONIC FATIGUE
AND
FIBROMYALGIA

DON COLBERT, M.D.

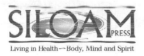

Living in Health—Body, Mind and Spirit

THE BIBLE CURE FOR CHRONIC FATIGUE AND
FIBROMYALGIA by Don Colbert, M.D.
Published by Siloam Press
A part of Strang Communications Company
600 Rinehart Road
Lake Mary, Florida 32746
www.siloampress.com

Fresh Hope
for a New You!

Physical and spiritual refreshment, vigor and joy will arm you against the symptoms of chronic fatigue syndrome and fibromyalgia! If you feel physically depleted and emotionally drained, God has good news for you. He has provided strength and power for your battle, and He will energize you as you take these natural and spiritual Bible Cure steps.

Jesus Christ promises you rest, refreshment, restoration and renewal. For He said, "Come to me, all of you who are weary and carry heavy burdens, and I will give you rest. Take my yoke upon you. Let me teach you, because I am humble and gentle, and you will find rest for your souls" (Matt. 11:28–29).

If you are often overwhelmed by fatigue that saps your strength and robs your life—fatigue that will simply not go away—then you are not alone. A recent study in *The Archives of Internal Medicine* has documented that over 800,000 people nationwide suffer from chronic fatigue syndrome. "For years, this medical condition has been marginalized and misunderstood," says Kim Kenney, executive director of The Chronic Fatigue and Immune Dysfunction Association of America.[1]

Many individuals with chronic fatigue also have fibromyalgia. In fibromyalgia, muscular skeletal pain accompanies chronic fatigue.

This Bible Cure booklet is dynamically packed with powerful information about natural and spiritual solutions to energize you to win the battle. Chronic fatigue and fibromyalgia are not God's plan for you, for God's mighty Word promises: "'For I know the plans I have for you,' says the LORD. 'They are plans for good and not for disaster, to give you a future and a hope. In those days when you pray, I will listen. If you look for me in earnest, you will find me when you seek me. I will be found by you'" (Jer. 29:11–14). So you see, God's desires that you conquer your fatigue and discover power and energy to live life to the fullest.

Be Encouraged and Energized!

So as you read this book, get ready to defeat the symptoms of chronic fatigue syndrome and fibromyalgia. You will begin to feel better physically, emotionally and spiritually. This Bible Cure booklet is filled with practical steps, hope, encouragement and valuable information on how to stay fit and healthy. In this book, you will

> *uncover God's divine plan of health*
> *for body, soul and spirit*
> *through modern medicine, good nutrition*
> *and the medicinal power*
> *of Scripture and prayer.*

You will discover life-changing and healing scriptures throughout this booklet that will strengthen and energize you.

As you read, apply and trust God's promises, you will also uncover powerful Bible Cure prayers to help you line up your thoughts and feelings with God's plan of divine health for you—a plan that includes living victoriously. In this Bible Cure booklet, you will be energized by the following chapters:

There is much you can do to prevent or overcome your symptoms. The Bible Cure plan will energize you with confidence, determination and knowledge to live victoriously. God's healing power is greater than any fatigue and pain that you now face.

You no longer have to be weary and burdened. The Bible Cure promise for you is this:

> He gives power to those who are tired and
> worn out; he offers strength to the weak.
> —Isaiah 40:29

It is my prayer that the power of faith in God's wonderful Word and the divine touch of His healing hand, together with practical suggestions for health, nutrition and fitness in this book, will restore your health, energy, vitality and joy!

—Don Colbert, M.D.

vii

A Bible Cure Prayer
FOR YOU

Almighty God, You are the source of all power and strength. You have said that You give Your people strength. So I ask You to break the spirit of heaviness and weariness in my body and give me the knowledge and wisdom to eat correctly and to live well. Help me overcome fatigue and pain and become energized to serve and worship You with my whole heart, mind, body and strength. Empower me to accomplish Your purpose and plans for my life. In You I will find my rest and strength. Amen.

Chapter 1

Know Your Enemy—
Understanding Chronic
Fatigue and Fibromyalgia

An ancient and powerful biblical proverb reads: "How useless to spread a net in full view of all the birds!" (Prov. 1:17, NIV). That means an enemy cannot win if you see and understand what he is doing. Your enemy is chronic fatigue syndrome, and according to the proverb, your first Bible Cure step to victory is to understand your condition.

Armed with a factual, truthful knowledge about what you are facing, you will better know how to pray and make wise treatment decisions. God does not intend for us to accept passively the physical attacks that assault us. We can fight back with knowledge, wisdom, faith and prayer! In the natural we can strengthen our immune systems, and in the spiritual realm, we can strengthen our faith.

1

Make this Bible Cure prayer your own as you read this chapter and develop both natural and spiritual insight about your condition:

> You are my strength; I wait for you to rescue me, for you, O God, are my place of safety . . . O my Strength, to you I sing praises, for you, O God, are my refuge, the God who shows me unfailing love. Amen.
> —PSALM 59:9, 17

Understanding the Battle

Chronic fatigue syndrome (CFS) is fatigue that is so severe it is disabling. When diagnosed in its early stages, chronic fatigue is much easier to treat.

There is no known cure for CFS, which also is called chronic fatigue, immune dysfunction syndrome (CFIDS). Symptoms include debilitating fatigue that is not improved by bed rest and may be worsened by physical or mental activity, impairment of short-term memory or concentration, sore throat, tender lymph nodes, muscle and joint pain and headaches. Symptoms must be present for more than six months without any other medical explanation. Individuals with CFS function at a substantially lower level of activity than before onset of the illness, and many continue holding jobs, attending school or caring for themselves or family members.[1]

Common Causes of Chronic Fatigue

1. Chronic candida (yeast) infections and other chronic infections often caused by the overuse of antibiotics, food allergies, anemia, low blood sugar and low thyroid function
2. Excessive stress
3. Sleep disturbances
4. Depression

Take this self-test to help assess whether or not you are experiencing the symptoms of chronic fatigue syndrome.

A BIBLE CURE HEALTH TIP

Has your activity level been reduced by 50 percent in the past six months because of fatigue that seemed to come on all at once? If other fatigue-causing illnesses have been factored out, this is the major criterion for diagnosing chronic fatigue syndrome. Check the common symptoms of chronic fatigue syndrome that you are experiencing. If you are experiencing eight of these minor criteria symptoms, then ask your doctor to examine you for chronic fatigue syndrome:

- ❏ Mild fever
- ❏ Recurrent sore throat
- ❏ Painful lymph nodes
- ❏ Muscle weakness
- ❏ Muscle pain
- ❏ Prolongued fatigue after exercise
- ❏ Recurrent headache
- ❏ Migratory joint pains
- ❏ Neurological or psychological complaints
- ❏ Sensitivity to bright light
- ❏ Forgetfulness
- ❏ Confusion
- ❏ Inability to concentrate
- ❏ Excessive irritability
- ❏ Depression
- ❏ Sleep disturbance (either sleeping too much or an inability to sleep)

If you are experiencing symptoms of chronic fatigue, get a complete physical exam by your medical doctor and a thorough evaluation by a nutritional doctor.

Your doctor will need to rule out a number of diseases that are also linked to excessive fatigue. In addition, chronic fatigue can also be a side effect of certain medications, including antihistamines, blood pressure medications, arthritis medications, antianxiety medications, tranquilizers, antidepressants and numerous other medications.

Fibromyalgia shares the same symptoms and remedies as chronic fatigue syndrome, but it has some additional factors as well. Let's take a look.

Fibromyalgia

Fibromyalgia is actually a rheumatic type of disorder characterized by diffuse muscular skeletal pain with trigger points, or tender points throughout the body, sleep disturbances and fatigue. Common associated symptoms include depression, irritable bowel, irritability, headaches, dizziness, decreased memory, temporal mandibular joint symptoms and anxiety.

If you are experiencing this condition, your fatigue is accompanied by extremely tender muscles, which usually occur in specific areas of the body. Nine different trigger points are commonly associated with fibromyalgia. These include the muscles in the neck, in the upper back, in the mid-back, at the base of the skull, in the buttocks, in the upper portion of the thigh, just above the lateral elbow and in the rib cage, especially around the second rib.

The major symptoms include:

- Six or more trigger points of the body that are reproducible

- Muscle aches, pains and stiffness of a minimum of three different areas for at least three months

Disorders that produce similar symptoms must be excluded. The minor symptoms include:

- Sleep disturbances
- Irritable bowel syndrome
- Generalized fatigue
- Chronic headache
- Tingling or numbing sensations
- Swelling of the joints
- Psychological and neurological complaints
- Symptoms varying in intensity with activity, stress or changes in weather

Fibromyalgia is much more common in women than in men. Some reports have said that it occurs as much as ten times more often in women than in men. Medical tests such as x-rays and blood tests usually do not reveal any abnormalities.

Getting Down to the Root Causes

When chronic candida infections, food allergies, excessive stress, sleep deprivation and depression take their toll on an individual's immune system, chronic fatigue syndrome (CFS) and fibromyalgia can result. Doctors commonly find a suppressed immune system and low adrenal function in their CFS patients. Let's take a closer look at the causes of chronic fatigue and fibromyalgia.

Candidiasis

A common cause of these diseases is prolonged candidiasis, commonly called yeast infection. *Candida albicans* is a yeast organism that has been around for thousands of years. This yeast is normally present in the gastrointestinal tracts of healthy people. Yeast is a single-celled organism that thrives on the surface of other living things, including our fruits, grains, vegetables and even our skin. Yeast is similar to fungus. Mushrooms, molds and mildew are all different types of yeast.

Candida yeast normally lives in the gastrointestinal tract and the vagina. It thrives among trillions of bacteria. Many of these good bacteria (called the lactobacillus) prevent the overgrowth of yeast, prevent buildup of disease-forming bacteria and even synthesize certain vitamins.

Only small numbers of yeast candida are normally present in our gastrointestinal tracts. The lactobacilli (good bacteria) balance the yeast so that they are unable to grow out of control. Our immune systems also help to keep the yeast in

7

check. However, when we take potent antibiotics, especially over a prolonged period of time, much of the good bacteria are destroyed and the critical balance of microorganisms in the gastrointestinal tract is upset. When too many of the lactobacilli have been killed, the yeast can grow unimpeded.

Other factors that can cause yeast overgrowth include cortisone, birth control pills, pregnancy, environmental chemicals, diabetes, certain foods (especially sugars) and allergies. Allergies and viral infections tend to drain the immune system. When the immune system is weakened, yeast is able to multiply unchecked. Deficiencies in digestive secretions can also lead to an overgrowth of candida. Pancreatic enzymes, hydrochloric acid and bile will help prevent the overgrowth of candida.

The Symptoms of Candidiasis

Candidiasis can cause impaired memory, distractability, irritability and agitation, inability to concentrate, feeling drunk without consuming alcohol, anxiety, depression and insomnia. Gastrointestinal symptoms include bloating, swelling, spastic colon, diarrhea, loud intestinal rumblings, cramping, excessive gas, itching of the anus, mucus in the stools and heartburn.

While these are the most common symptoms of candidiasis that I see, candidiasis can also affect nearly every system of the body, including the immune system, endocrine system and the genito-urinary system.

Too Much of a Good Thing

I see cases of candidiasis on a daily basis in my practice, and I believe most of it is caused by the overuse of antibiotics. Decades ago, when anti biotics were first used they could kill almost any form of bacteria. However, bacteria have changed their genetic makeup and have become increasingly resistant to the antibiotics. Now, resistant bacteria have become stronger and stronger, so that some strands of bacteria may be resistant to almost all forms of antibiotics.

While I am not against the use of antibiotics, for they have saved countless lives, I do believe they should be used sparingly. Many physicians prescribe them for flus and colds, although we know that antibiotics do not kill viruses. Some patients believe that antibiotics are good for all infections and often pressure their physicians to prescribe them. The extended use of antibiotics for treating acne, chronic sinus infections and chronic prostate infections will likely create a new disease that very few people are aware of: chronic candidiasis! Do you have it?[2]

Yeast

Candidiasis yeast will actually compete with the body for nutrition and rob it of nutrients. It releases toxic by-products such as alcohol, acetaldehyde and as many as seventy-nine different toxins that can circulate through the blood stream and affect other organs and tissues. This places a tremendous burden on the immune system. A viscous cycle of continual and progressive draining of the immune system begins.

In addition, the inflammation in the gastrointestinal tract creates a "leaky gut" in which food proteins and other foreign substances are able to travel directly into the circulatory system, triggering allergies and sensitivities in our bodies. This is one of the reasons why so many patients with chronic candidiasis develop severe food allergies and inhalant allergies. This cycle causes additional fatigue, and thus the cycle continues.

Candidiasis is only one cause of chronic fatigue and fibromyalgia. Stress is another culprit.

Stress and Fatigue

If you keep the headlights of your car on all night, the battery will run down. At first, you will be able to restart the car by jump-starting it. But if you leave the lights on continually night after night, eventually the battery will be so depleted that jump-starting it won't help.

The same thing occurs in our bodies with excessive stress. We stress our bodies with our fast-paced lifestyles, juggling demanding jobs with even more demanding family responsibilities. Daily we dodge traffic jams, race to prepare dinner and jog through malls and grocery stores to shop. Our schedules can leave us overworked, overwhelmed, spent and exhausted.

As you rush through your mornings, do you gulp down a cup of coffee with a doughnut, trying to get an energy jump-start? Year after year of stressful living and "jump-starting" the body daily with caffeinated beverages and high-sugar foods will eventually leave the body depleted.

As a family practitioner, most of my regular patients complain of too much stress. Stress that persists for years and decades will eventually drain the adrenal glands and leave us tired, run down and chronically fatigued.

Stress and Our Adrenal Glands

The adrenal glands are two very small glands about the size of the thumb that sit on top of the kidneys. These small glands are actually responsible for giving us the stamina to withstand the stresses of everyday life. An adrenal gland is divided into two parts and can be compared to a golf ball. The outer shell is the cortex. The adrenal cortex produces a number of different hormones, but the most important ones are cortisol and DHEA. Cortisol is very similar to the cortisone drugs, such as prednisone. The adrenal medulla is the central part of the adrenal gland, similar to the core of a golf ball. It secretes adrenaline.

When Our Reserves Run Dry

The body responds to emotional and physical stress as it would to a physical crisis. When you are faced with sudden danger, the adrenal medulla releases adrenaline for extra strength and energy. In other words, your "fight or flight" response empowers you to either fight the battle or flee.

For instance, if you were backpacking in the wilderness and stumbled upon a grizzly bear, you probably would not stand and fight the bear. Most likely you would flee. Adrenaline would shoot through your body, giving you nearly superhuman energy to help you escape from the bear.

With extreme stress, our bodies pump out potent chemicals that get us ready for fight or flight. But in modern society, we face emotional and physical stress every day, and these high-energy chemicals needed for fight or flight are being released into our bodies continually. In addition, when we are sitting in our boss's office or in traffic, we can neither fight nor flee. Nevertheless, these chemicals are still released.

> *So don't worry about having enough food or drink or clothing. Why be like the pagans who are so deeply concerned about these things? Your heavenly Father already knows all your needs, and he will give you all you need from day to day if you live for him and make the Kingdom of God your primary concern.*
> MATTHEW 6:31 33

When stress responses are released continually into our bodies throughout the day for low-energy needs, we Americans can end up stewing in our own juices. Eventually, we will become physically and emotionally burned out. Our batteries will become depleted by using our adrenaline on low-energy needs—just like the car with its lights left on.

Food Allergies

Food allergies can also cause adrenal stress. Therefore, I suggest a comprehensive food allergy or food sensitivity test in order to determine the foods to which you are allergic.

Chronic Survival Response

The alarm reaction is only one response of the adrenal gland. The other is the long-term chronic survival response. This response is simply the body's long-term response to loss of control. Long-term loss of control leads to elevation of the adrenal cortex hormone *cortisol.* How many Americans dislike their jobs and feel trapped with the total loss of control over their futures? As a result of this feeling over an extended period of time, cortisol levels gradually rise.

Cortisol has different actions from the adrenaline released in the acute alarm response. This is a slower, more insidious process resulting in the following: blood pressure rises slowly, sodium is retained, gastric acids increase, sex hormones decrease, fats and clotting factors in the blood increase and the immune response is lowered.

This chronic survival response actually causes the body to be aroused in order to survive over a long period of time.

The chronic survival response leads to passivity and feelings of fail-

> *You will keep in perfect peace all who trust in you, whose thoughts are fixed on you! Trust in the LORD always, for the LORD GOD is the eternal Rock.*
> —Isaiah 26:3

ure and self-doubt. Eventually it can lead to depression and chronic fatigue. Conversely, the alarm response is usually active, releasing anger, hostility, aggression or verbal outbursts. The chronic survival response is passive, and feelings and emotions are actually not released but are turned inward. This is similar to an animal that, when faced by a larger animal, may play dead in order to survive.

Alarm reactions may occur up to fifty to a hundred times a day depending on the stress the individual is under. However, the chronic survival response is simply a mind-set of chronic loss of control. A mother who worries about her teenage daughter who has run away from home may experience it. A businessman in middle management who sees no way of ever being promoted or the wife of an alcoholic husband who sees no way out of her predicament may also be experiencing this response. Such individuals may begin to drag themselves through their days, exhausted and lethargic. They are chronically fatigued.

Stress is harmful to the body in so many different ways. Stress can seriously affect your ability to sleep at night, in addition to other sleep disturbances, which is another major cause of chronic fatigue syndrome and fibromyalgia.

Sleep Disturbances

Sleep disturbances and depression are the most common causes of these diseases that I see in my practice.

Normal sleep actually occurs in cycles, with the average person experiencing about five or six sleep cycles during a normal night's sleep. Each sleep cycle typically lasts about sixty to ninety minutes. The first part of the cycle is composed of four stages. The deeper stages, stages three and four, are the more restful part of sleep. Stages one and two are more superficial sleep.

The second part of the cycle is the rapid eye movement, or the REM phase of sleep. During this phase of sleep, dreaming occurs. The majority of the time in the first ninety-minute cycle is spent in the first phase of the cycle, including the four stages, and only minutes are spent in the second phase of the REM cycle.

However, with each successive ninety-minute sleep cycle, less time is spent in phase one and more time is spent in phase two. In the final ninety-minute sleep cycle, before awakening in the morning, REM sleep takes up the majority of the time of the cycle, and only a few minutes are spent in phase one. Thus, many times before awakening, many people can remember their dreams.

Those who awaken during the transition from phase one to REM sleep are often very tired when they awaken in the morning, and thus they are very fatigued throughout the day. A variety of sleeping disorders, which we will discuss in greater depth later on, can interrupt sleep and eventually trigger a pattern of chronic fatigue.

Your Fatigue

You've probably realized by now that chronic fatigue is not a simple disease. Many factors, or a combination of factors, may be responsible for your fatigue. As we have discussed some major causes of chronic fatigue and fibromyalgia, have you seen your own symptoms? Throughout the rest of this booklet I will be providing natural and spiritual remedies that will arm you to battle your enemy and defeat chronic fatigue and fibromyalgia and their symptoms forever!

God's Plan for You

As I stated at the beginning of this booklet, God's plan for your life is only good—filled with good events, prosperity, health and uplifting relationships. But to experience His plan, you need energy and strength.

Start getting energized daily by reading God's Word and praying. Let your desire echo the words of King David, "My life is an example to many, because you have been my strength and protection" (Ps. 71:7).

Claim the promise of God's strength and protection throughout your days. Read the scriptures in this booklet and memorize them. Use them as spiritual medicine for your soul. Pray the Bible Cure prayers as you connect to God's power and energy for your life.

A BIBLE CURE PRAYER
FOR YOU

When I think of the wisdom and scope of God's plan, I fall to my knees and pray to the Father, the Creator of everything in heaven and on earth. I pray that from His glorious, unlimited resources He will give me mighty inner strength through His Holy Spirit. And I pray that Christ will be more and more at home in my heart as I trust in Him. May my roots go down deep into the soil of God's marvelous love. And may I have the power to understand, as all God's people should, how wide, how long, how high and how deep His love for me really is. May I experience the love of Christ, though it is so great I will never fully understand it. Then I will be filled with the fullness of life and power that comes from God. Now glory be to God! By His mighty power at work within me, He is able to accomplish infinitely more than I would ever dare to ask or hope. Amen.

—Adapted from Ephesians 3:14–20

19

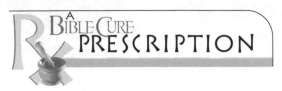

A BIBLE CURE PRESCRIPTION

Trust God daily to renew your strength and energize you as you pray and read His Word. Check anything that may be causing fatigue in your lifestyle:

- ❏ Sleep disturbances
- ❏ Excessive stress, leading to low adrenal function and eventually to adrenal exhaustion
- ❏ Chronic candida (yeast) infections due to a suppressed immune system
- ❏ Food sensitivities and food allergies
- ❏ Depression
- ❏ Other: _____

Write a prayer asking for God's help in applying the knowledge and wisdom you will learn in this booklet to energize you in overcoming these causes of fatigue:

_____

_____

_____

_____

Chapter 2

Refuel
With Nutrition

The Bible Cure for you to be energized and overcome chronic fatigue begins with good nutrition. You wouldn't put water into your gas tank and expect your car to run, would you? Your car needs to be fueled properly, according to its design. Well, the designer of your body, God, has provided just the right fuel for you!

> And God said, "Look! I have given you the seed-bearing plants throughout the earth and all the fruit trees for your food. And I have given all the grasses and other green plants to the animals and birds for their food." And so it was. Then God looked over all he had made, and he saw that it was excellent in every way.
>
> —GENESIS 1:29–31

As a foundation in overcoming chronic fatigue and fibromyalgia and being energized to enjoy life, I strongly recommend that you follow the Balanced Carb-Protein-Fat Plan found in my book *Walking in Divine Health.* This diet will benefit you greatly, no matter what the root cause of your chronic fatigue. If your diet contains excessive sugar, fat, starch and salt, you are probably experiencing fatigue and even chronic fatigue. Balanced nutrition helps your body fight off fatigue and sustains you through demanding and stressful situations.

Overcoming Candidiasis

If your symptoms are caused by yeast infections, prolonged use of antibiotics or by food allergies, a specialized diet for three to six months will change your life completely.

Cookies, candies, cakes, pies and soft drinks will feed candidiasis to the point at which the yeast grows out of control. Changing your diet is the most important thing you can do to begin treating chronic candidiasis. Start by avoiding, eliminating or radically reducing the following:

1. **All sweets.** Sweets include white sugar (sucrose, fructose, glucose,

galactose and sorbitol) and all other sugars, including corn syrup, dextrose, barley malt, honey, molasses, brown rice syrup and even fruit juice. Avoid all pastries, breads and other bakery goods containing yeast.

2. **Milk products.** Milk and all milk products should be restricted. The sugar in milk, which is lactose, actually feeds the yeast, as does regular sugar. Milk protein is also one of the most common food allergies. It can further weaken your immune system, thus encouraging candida overgrowth. Cheeses should be avoided because they contain yeast or mold, and blue cheese, or Roquefort, is one of the worst. You should also avoid fermented dairy products such as yogurt, buttermilk and sour cream, since these products contain yeast.

3. **Vinegar.** Foods containing vinegar, such as soy sauce, barbecue sauce, steak sauce, mustard, ketchup, mayonnaise, salad dressings, horseradish and pickled vegetables should be avoided because they contain yeast.

(Note: If you cannot limit or avoid yeast- and mold-containing foods, you should at least avoid sugary foods such as cakes, pies, candy, colas and pastries.)

4. **Meats that have been processed or smoked should also be avoided.** These include bacon, sausage, ham, smoked turkey and other processed meats.

5. **Dried fruits,** including raisins, figs and dates, should also be avoided.

6. **Coffee.** Limit or avoid drinking coffee completely.

7. **Peanuts and peanut butter** should be avoided since they commonly contain mold.

8. **Melons.** Limit or avoid most melons, especially cantaloupe.

9. **All alcoholic beverages,** including beer, wine and mixed drinks, should be avoided since they contain extremely high amounts of yeast along with simple carbohydrates that feed yeast.

10. **Food allergens.** The next category of foods to avoid are food allergens,

or foods that tend to cause allergies. Most people with candidiasis have many food allergies. The most common ones are eggs, milk, wheat and corn. However, in order to determine which foods you are allergic or sensitive to, have a food allergy test such as the ELISA Test or the ALCAT.

11. **Starchy grains and vegetables.** Finally, it is best to limit your intake of starchy grains and vegetables, including beans, peas, potatoes, sweet potatoes, corn, oats, wheat and pasta. Some good grain alternatives are buckwheat, amaranth, quinoa, millet and brown rice. Before cooking rice, it is best to soak it in water for several hours, then drain it and rinse it. This will remove enzyme inhibitors from the outer husks of the rice.

Try to avoid both yeast- and mold containing foods as much as possible. However, yeast- and mold-containing foods such as breads, enriched flour, alcoholic beverages, vinegar, aged cheeses, fermented dairy products, mushrooms, peanut butter, coffee and canned juices do not actually make candida grow. When people develop symptoms from eating yeast- or mold-containing foods, it's usually because they are allergic to the yeast.

Leftovers may contain mold, too. I'm sure that you've noticed how green mold grows on cheese that has been left sitting in the refrigerator opened for a few weeks.

But remember, the main foods that make yeast or candida grow are high-sugar foods! Sugar-containing foods are the main nutrients for yeast. These include not only simple sugars such as sucrose, fructose, corn syrup, honey, fruit juice and maple syrup, but also even milk and dairy products. Milk sugar is called lactose. This also causes excessive yeast overgrowth.

What Can I Eat?

To simplify things, I will list the following food groups that you may freely enjoy while you are on the candida diet.

Meat and fish proteins. These include chicken, lean beef (preferably free-range), veal, turkey, wild game, lamb and pork. (Pork is forbidden in the Book of Leviticus in the Bible, but if you must eat it, be sure it is very lean.) Also included in the list of protein foods are shellfish, including shrimp, lobster, crab and so forth. (All varieties of shellfish are also forbidden in Leviticus under ancient Judaic law.) Herring, salmon, mackerel, tuna and most other fish are recommended as long as they are not breaded.

Vegetables. Low-starch vegetables include broccoli, Brussels sprouts, celery, cabbage, cauliflower, carrots, collard greens and eggplant. Leafy greens include lettuce, spinach, parsley, collard greens, beet greens, watercress, kale, chard (mustard greens), onions, bell peppers, snow peas, string beans, tomatoes, turnips, eggplant and artichokes.

Grains and nuts. These include amaranth, quinoa, millet and buckwheat. Nuts and seeds include almonds, flaxseeds, sunflower seeds, pumpkin seeds, pecans and Brazil nuts. Nuts are difficult for many people to digest. Therefore, I recommend that you soak them in filtered or distilled water overnight for at least twelve hours, preferably in a glass container or jar. Drain the water and store the nuts in the refrigerator in an airtight container. This causes the nuts to sprout, which makes them easier to digest.

Oils. Organic, unrefined vegetable oils, butter, organic butter and extra-virgin olive oil are permitted. The unrefined vegetable oils include sunflower oil, safflower oil, pumpkin seed oil and flaxseed oil. Unrefined oils are best used in salad dressings. Cook with either organic butter or olive oil.

Margarine and all refined oils, such as oils found in grocery stores, should be eliminated from the diet. Margarine and refined oils can contribute to a variety of degenerative diseases.

Starchy vegetables. For the first three to four weeks, avoid starchy vegetables including potatoes, sweet potatoes, lentils, peas, beans and other legumes, rice, corn, pasta, popcorn, crackers, cereals, pancakes, waffles, muffins, tortillas, wheat, oats, rye, barley, spelt and artichokes. Afterward you may start eating more of the starchy vegetables. If you are sensitive to wheat products and if they cause you bloating, gas or a lot of rumbling in your stomach, then I recommend that you avoid wheat bread, wheat crackers, pasta, pancakes and waffles.

Liver Detoxification

Excessive yeast overgrowth is often linked with too many toxins (or poisons) in the liver. If you are experiencing constant yeast infections, you may need to undergo a nutritional program to detox your liver. Detoxifying the liver can be extremely important in overcoming severe candidiasis.

The liver purifies the body of substances such as drugs, alcohol and other chemicals by combining them with a nutrient, which then converts them to a less toxic substance.

The two phases of detoxification of the liver are referred to as *phase one* and *phase two detoxification*. However, the intermediate products between phase one and phase two may be very toxic to the body until they are neutralized. Nutrients that help to detoxify the liver include milk thistle, silymarin, black currant oil, lipoic acid, DL methionine, phosphatidyl choline, beet root and garlic. Many other herbs and nutrients also aid in the detoxification of the liver.

Contact your nutritional physician to determine if you should take this step, and undergo liver detoxification under his or her supervision.

Speaking Frankly About Fiber

Many individuals don't get enough fiber and water in their diets—and chronic constipation is the unpleasant result. In order to clear yeast from the GI (gastrointestinal) tract, it's important to have regular bowel movements—at least one every day. Enjoy lots of raw vegetables in your diet, and drink at least two quarts of water a day.

Fiber binds yeast and prevents it from being reabsorbed in the body. You may also consider taking a fiber supplement, such as freshly ground flaxseeds. Take 5 teaspoons per day. You may also take rice bran, microcrystalline cellulose or psyllium. Psyllium fiber supplements are commonly sold over the counter. Take one that does not contain sugar or NutraSweet. Perdiem Fiber is a good one, and you can find it at the grocery store.

The Good Guys

As I have already mentioned, getting rid of bad bacteria with antibiotics can cause the good guys, or the good bacteria, to be killed off too. Without the good guys, yeast grows wild.

Billions of these good bacteria live in our intestinal tract and keep the intestines clean by feeding on the waste, fungus, yeast and other harmful bacteria. The good guys also produce vitamins, hormones and proteins that our bodies need.

Therefore, during the process of clearing yeast from the body, you need to take in good bacteria so that the bowel will be recolonized with it.

I recommend approximately three to six billion colony-forming units of lactobacillus acidophilus and lactobacillus bifidus. There are other good forms of bacteria, including *Lactobacillus Plantarum, Lactobacillus Salavarius* and *Lactobacillus Sporogenes*. You may be thinking, *Where on earth do I find this?* You can find the "good bacteria" in capsules or powder form at the health food store. It may be called Probiotics or Intestinal Flora.

> *My health may fail, and my spirit may grow weak, but God remains the strength of my heart; he is mine forever.*
> —PSALM 73:26

Livestock and Antibiotics

Did you realize that much of the meat we eat every day is loaded with antibiotics? "About one-quarter of the antibiotics used in the United States each year—some nineteen million pounds—are given to livestock. Some 60 to 80 percent of all cattle, sheep, swine and poultry in the United States will be given antibiotics at some point. The 30 different antibiotics are given in so-called subtherapeutic amounts—doses lower than those needed to treat specific diseases."[1]

Every time you eat a steak or a chicken thigh, you are ingesting antibiotics. These antibiotics are killing off the beneficial bacteria in our bodies and making us increasingly prone to getting candidiasis. It's critically important to take in good bacteria daily to replace what's being destroyed by the antibiotics in the meat that we eat.

Get Started!

Since chronic fatigue and fibromyalgia may range from mild tiredness to extreme exhaustion to distressing muscle pain, it is best to seek nutritional treatment early. The longer it persists, the longer it takes to turn the problem around. Make a decision to start eating for energy right now.

Conclusion

Whether your chronic fatigue and fibromyalgia are caused by yeast, allergies, antibiotics or any of the other culprits that may be taxing your immune system and stealing your energy, the first place to go for answers is always Jesus Christ. He understands your body, for He created it. And He loves and understands you. And just as every good father wants the best for his children, He longs for you to experience a richer, more abundant life.

Have you ever used sugar or breads and pastries to fill a physical or even an emotional void? Sugar is not the source of your power or energy

> *Give all your worries and cares to God, for he cares about what happens to you.*
> —1 PETER 5:7

in life—God is. In fact, the Bible says that the bread of life is Jesus Himself. Your dependence on yeast products in the natural may be robbing you of a more important spiritual focus in your life—Jesus Christ, the bread of life.

If you have a dependence on bread and yeast or sugar products in your life, then turn to the true bread of life as your source. When you become hungry for bread, remember His promise to you: "I am the bread of life. No one who comes to me will ever be hungry again. Those who believe in me will never thirst" (John 6:35).

A BIBLE CURE PRAYER
FOR YOU

Lord Jesus, break any dependence I have on natural bread and fill my hunger for bread with Your living bread. Help me to discern how dependent I am on sugar and yeast products. Give me the strength and will power to eliminate these products from my life and to feed on Your bread and drink Your living water. Amen.

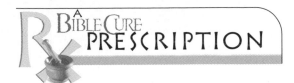

A Bible Cure PRESCRIPTION

What products do you need to eliminate from your diet?

_____

_____

Describe how dependent you are on sugar:

_____

_____

List the healthy foods you will include in your diet:

_____

_____

Write a prayer asking God to free you from any dependence you may have on sugar or yeast products.

_____

_____

_____

_____

Chapter 3

Recharge
With Exercise

The apostle Paul said, "I discipline my body like an athlete, training it to do what it should. Otherwise, I fear that after preaching to others I myself might be disqualified" (1 Cor. 9:27). Like the apostle Paul, I believe in the powerful benefits of exercise. Regular, daily exercise can help to eliminate the affects of stress, which is another major cause of chronic fatigue and fibromyalgia.

Guitar Strings

You cannot live in this world without experiencing stress. I have heard an expression that finding the right amount of stress is like tuning the strings of a guitar. If they are too tight, they may break. However, if they are too loose, you may not enjoy the music. You may be surprised to discover that you've been experiencing much more stress than you thought.

How much stress are you experiencing right now? Take this stress test to get in touch with the current level of stress in your life.

Are You Stressed Out? Your Stress Scale

Look up stress-producing changes in your life in the following table and see how stressed out you really are. Add up your score of the stressful events you have experienced over the past twelve months.

	STRESS	EVENT VALUES
1.	Death of spouse	100
2.	Divorce	60
3.	Menopause	60
4.	Separation from a partner	60
5.	Jail term or probation	60
6.	Death of a close family member other than spouse	60
7.	Serious personal injury or illness	45
8.	Marriage or establishing life partnership	45
9.	Fired at work	45
10.	Marital or relationship reconciliation	40
11.	Retirement	40
12.	Change in health of an immediate family member	40

If your total stress score over the last twelve months is 250 or greater, you may be feeling over-stressed, even if you are normally stress tolerant. Persons with a low tolerance for stress may be overstressed at levels beginning at 150.

Exercise can help you to overcome the fatigue caused by excessive stress over a long period of time. Following are some steps you can take to help overcome fatigue with exercise.

Breathing Exercises

Practice abdominal breathing. Resting or relaxing during the day without taking a nap is also very beneficial for relieving stress. When you are resting or relaxing, you may want to listen to a relaxation tape or calm, soothing music and practice deep breathing exercises. Abdominal breathing, which involves moving the abdominal muscles outward, has been shown to be the best form of breathing to relieve stress. Chest breathing tends to be more shallow and rapid and is commonly practiced when a person is under stress.

Many trained singers and musicians are abdominal breathers. However, the majority of people are chest breathers. In order to learn abdominal breathing, it is best to lie on your back and place a large book on the abdomen, such as a dictionary or a large family Bible. While breathing, move the abdomen outward, thus causing the book to rise higher in the air. Concentrate on moving the abdomen outward and not expanding the rib cage.

> *But the seventh day is a day of rest dedicated to the LORD your God. On that day no one in your household may do any kind of work. This includes you, your sons and daughters, your male and female servants, your livestock, and any foreigners living among you. For in six days the LORD made the heavens, the earth, the sea, and everything in them; then he rested on the seventh day. That is why the LORD blessed the Sabbath day and set it apart as holy.*
> —EXODUS 20:10–11

As this is practiced, you will be able to perform abdominal breathing while sitting, standing or walking. When you feel stressed, perform five or ten slow, deep, abdominal breaths to relax your body.

Progressive Muscle Relaxation Exercises

Practice this when you are reclining in a comfortable chair, on a bed or on the couch. Close your eyes to relax. Beginning with the feet, tense the toes by curling them under; hold this position for five seconds and then relax. As you relax, simply let the tension leave your body.

Next, flex the ankle joint. Pull the toes back while flexing the calf muscle. Again, hold this position for five seconds and then relax. Next, point the toes like a ballerina, and again flex the calf for five seconds. Move to the legs and flex the thighs tight. Hold this for five seconds and relax.

Gradually working your way up your body, flex the muscles in the abdomen, arms, chest, shoulders, hands, neck, forehead, eyes and jaw. Once again, do each of these for five seconds and then relax. The tension will actually melt away.

Develop a Regular Exercise Program

Nothing is more invigorating than practicing a

regular exercise routine. You may feel too exhausted to even think about jogging at this point, but what about walking? Brisk walking is the best exercise to start with. You should walk fast enough so that you cannot sing, yet slowly enough so that you can talk. Start slowly, and gradually build your exercise routine. Do something you love. If you love the outdoors, take a brisk walk through your favorite park. If a busy city street stimulates you, walk to your favorite florist and buy yourself a fresh flower each day, or to your favorite newsstand to purchase a sports magazine.

Here are some tips for staying with it. Don't look at exercise as something you can do in your spare time. Make

> *The LORD gives his people strength. The LORD blesses them with peace.*
> —PSALM 29:11

this time an important part of your day. In addition, don't think about it as work. See it as a special time to be alone with God, surrounded by the wonders of His creation. As you exercise, thank God for all of His love for you and for His blessings in your life.

Begin this daily walking program. Before long, you may begin to wonder where all of your stress went.

A Simple Walking Program

(NOTE: Each column indicates the number of minutes to walk. Complete three exercise sessions each week. If you find a particular week's pattern tiring, repeat it before going on to the next pattern. You do not have to complete the walking program in twelve weeks.)

Week	—Walk	—Walk Briskly	—Walk	—Minutes
1	5	5	5	15
2	5	7	5	17
3	5	9	5	19
4	5	11	5	21
5	5	13	5	23
6	5	15	5	25
7	5	18	5	28
8	5	20	5	30
9	5	23	5	33
10	5	26	5	36
11	5	28	5	38
12	5	30	5	40

Week 13 and thereafter: Check your pulse periodically to see if you are exercising within your target zone. As you get more in shape, try exercising within the upper range of your target zone. Gradually increase your brisk walking time to 30 to 60 minutes, three or four times a week. Remember that your goal is to get the benefits you are seeking and enjoy your activity.

A Word of Caution

If you have been under continual, chronic stress for many years and feel totally exhausted, you may have a very low adrenal function. If simple brisk walking causes exhaustion, then you should refrain from doing this form of exercise until your adrenal function has been restored. Rest and take the supplements that will be discussed in chapter 5 to restore adrenal function. By following the other Bible Cure steps to restore adrenal function you will eventually be able to perform moderate exercise without exhaustion.

Never push yourself if you feel exhausted after exercise. You could further weaken your adrenal glands and cause even more severe fatigue. Use balance and wisdom.

Ready for More?

Your fatigue may not be at such a severe level. If so, you may be able to skip the earlier building stages and get into more vigorous exercise. Aerobic exercise, such as brisk walking, swimming or cycling, will usually improve the quality of sleep. Regular aerobic exercise helps the body to make smooth transitions between sleep cycles and stages of sleep. Exercise for twenty to thirty minutes a day at

65 to 80 percent of your predicted maximal heart rate. To determine your training heart rate, see the chart below.

Your Predicted Heart Rate

Calculate your target heart zone using this formula:

220 minus [your age] = _____
x .65 = _____
[This is your minimum.]

220 minus [your age] = _____
x .80 = _____
[This is your maximum.]

This example may help: To calculate the target heart zone for a 40-year-old man, subtract the age (40) from 220 (220- 40–180). Multiply 180 by .65, which equals 117. Then multiply 180 by .80, which equals 144. A 40-year old man's target heart rate zone is 117–144 beats per minute.

Conclusion

With God's help in taking these simple, practical steps, you can reduce stress and its accompanying fatigue while increasing strength and vitality. If you find yourself under constant stress in the world's fast-paced system, then take comfort in this Bible Cure promise: "For this Good News—that God has prepared a place of rest—has been announced to us just as it was to them" (Heb. 4:2). Rest isn't just for individuals who lived during Bible times. God's rest is for you right now.

A BIBLE CURE PRAYER
FOR YOU

Heavenly Father, help me reduce the stress in my life that robs my vitality and saps my strength. Show me how to work with more wisdom instead of working in ways that foolishly waste my strength. Fill me with Your peace and rest so that I may be renewed by Your presence and power. Thank You for giving me the peace that passes all understanding. Amen.

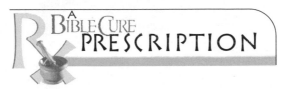

A BIBLE CURE PRESCRIPTION

Check the ways you will begin reducing your stress:

- ❏ Regular exercise
- ❏ Practicing abdominal breathing
- ❏ Using muscle relaxation exercises
- ❏ List the things you plan to thank God for today as you start your exercise program:

_____

_____

_____

_____

_____

_____

_____

_____

Chapter 4

Renew With Rest

God plans to renew you, strengthen you and refresh you with rest. If you feel completely drained, tired and spent, you may have some doubts about that. Stop looking at the enormity of your fatigue and begin seeing the greatness of God.

Consider God's promise to you:

> Have you never heard or understood? Don't you know that the LORD is the ever-lasting God, the Creator of all the earth? He never grows faint or weary. No one can measure the depths of his understanding. He gives power to those who are tired and worn out; he offers strength to the weak. Even youths will become exhausted, and young men will give up. But those who

wait on the LORD will find new strength.
They will fly high on wings like eagles.
They will run and not grow weary. They
will walk and not faint.

—ISAIAH 40:28–31

This promise is for you. You will run and not be weary when you put your trust in God. What a wonderful promise, and what a wonderful God! He is so great that He created the universe, but is greater still because He sees you, right there in your circumstances, and He cares for you with a love that knows no limits. He will get you through this, and you will feel good once more. Isn't that great news?

Are You Getting Your Rest?

My son plays golf, however, he often forgets to charge his golf cart. On his way to the golf course, the golf cart suddenly runs out of juice, and he is left having to push it back home in order to charge it. Our bodies are very similar. If we do not adequately recharge our bodies with enough deep, restful sleep, our minds and our bodies will become extremely fatigued and will burn out before the end of the day.

During sleep, our bodies are repairing tissues that have been damaged or excessively stressed during the waking hours of the day. When you do not rest properly, your body becomes fatigued very quickly.

While many people do not know how much sleep they actually need, most need, on average, about seven to eight hours every night. Some people, however, may manage on just five or six hours, while others may need as many as ten hours of sleep a night.

Women usually need to sleep longer than men. Elderly patients usually sleep less as they age. However, they still require about seven to eight hours of sleep a night. Often the reduction in sleep experienced by the elderly is because the sleep hormone, melatonin, decreases with age.

Our bodies need sleep to resist disease, maintain strength and endurance, increase vitality, improve our moods and even to slow down aging. Deep, restful sleep and adequate dreaming will fully restore our bodies and our brains, thus improving our intellectual abilities, our moods, our emotional strength and even our attitudes.

God is able to give you rest and restore your strength when you are weary. He will also help you discover the cause of your sleeplessness. Even if you are experiencing mild or severe depression, which can cause countless sleepless nights, the Bible cure will help. A number of natural ways for you to rest and overcome fatigue are available to you. Let me explore those ways with you.

Avoid Sleeping Pills

When individuals have trouble falling asleep or staying asleep, often they go to their doctor to get some sleeping pills. But did you know that many sleeping pills, especially benzodiazepines, actually tend to disrupt normal sleep? Sleeping pills interrupt the natural REM sleep cycle we spoke of earlier, as well as the deeper stages of non-REM sleep.

Therefore, sleeping pills can only help you receive very superficial sleep. You may get more hours of sleep, but you will still never enter the deeper stages of sleep. You will wake up groggy and will feel fatigued throughout the day.

Over-the-counter sleep medications and medications containing antihistamines, such as Benadryl, also commonly cause fatigue throughout the day.

Insomnia is simply difficulty falling asleep or difficulty staying asleep. Doctors think of it in terms of sleep-onset insomnia (difficulty falling asleep) and sleep-maintenance insomnia (difficulty staying

51

there). The most common causes of sleep-onset insomnia are stress, anxiety, caffeine, alcohol, pain or discomfort or change in environment. Common causes of sleep-maintenance insomnia include depression, low blood sugar, nocturnal leg cramps, pain, alcohol and changes in environment.

Eliminate Stimulants

An important step in getting a good night's sleep is eliminating stimulants such as caffeine, decongestants and diet pills. These drugs will alter the normal architecture of sleep, preventing you from reaching the deep stages of sleep. They will also alter rapid eye movements, which will decrease your dreaming, cause fragmented sleep and increase fatigue.

Since a good night's sleep is probably the single most important factor in preventing fatigue, you should avoid or decrease substances that cause insomnia! Caffeine is a powerful stimulant, a drug that provides the body with no nutritional value at all. Caffeine arouses the body and actually activates the nerves and muscles. Caffeine is found in coffee, tea, soft drinks, chocolate, hot chocolate, certain medications and even coffee-flavored ice cream.

Caffeine

- The average amount of caffeine in a cup of coffee ranges from approximately 100–150 milligrams.
- The average amount of caffeine in a 12-ounce glass of tea is 70 milligrams.
- 7-Up, Sprite and most clear soft drinks have no caffeine.
- Mountain Dew has approximately 55 milligrams of caffeine.
- Coke has approximately 45 milligrams of caffeine.
- Pepsi has approximately 38 milligrams of caffeine.
- Jolt has approximately 100 milligrams of caffeine.

Caffeine will actually block the effects of serotonin and melatonin, which are two very important chemicals in the brain that cause you to fall asleep and remain asleep. If you are having difficulty sleeping, the first thing you should do is stop taking in caffeine.

Avoid Alcohol

Alcohol is another chemical that can cause major sleep disturbances. Many people think that a glass of wine at night will help relax them and help them fall asleep. Alcohol actually causes our bodies to release adrenaline, which gets us ready for "fight or flight," therefore stimulating our bodies.

Alcohol decreases tryptophan levels in the brain, which leads to lower serotonin levels and, as a result, causes sleep disturbances. Alcohol will also delay and actually decrease the REM stage of sleep, causing a person to sleep lightly and feel tired and groggy during the day.

Early to Bed

Do you go to bed after the evening news near midnight, after first falling asleep in front of the television set? Break late night habits. Go to bed as early in the evening as possible, and strive to get at least eight hours of sleep each night. Establish a regular bedtime. If an afternoon nap interferes with your sleep at night, then you should stop taking it.

Restless Leg Syndrome

Restless leg syndrome is another cause of chronic

fatigue. It is closely related to nocturnal myoclonus. Restless leg syndrome is simply that: restlessness of the legs. During sleep, this individual has a strong urge to move his legs. Nocturnal myoclonus is characterized by jerking movements or muscle contractions of leg muscles while asleep. The restless legs and contractions and cramping and jerking of the leg muscles may happen frequently throughout the night, causing insomnia and sleep disturbances that eventually result in extreme fatigue and exhaustion.

An iron deficiency can contribute to restless leg syndrome. Rule this out by getting your doctor to test your serum ferritin level, which measures how much iron your body has stored.

Muscle Cramps

If in addition to restless legs you also experience muscle cramps, especially in the calves, you may well have nocturnal myoclonus. If you are experiencing nocturnal myoclonus, take two tablets of chelated calcium and magnesium at bedtime at a dosage of 400 milligrams of calcium and 200 milligrams of magnesium. If you are over forty-five years old and have restless legs and muscle cramps in the calves, take 100 milligrams of ginkgo biloba three times a day as well. Be sure that you are getting enough vitamin E by taking 800 I.U.s a day.

If the above measures fail to relieve the symptoms of restless legs or muscle cramps in the calves, ask your physician to recommend either a sleep study or medication to increase dopamine, which usually relieves the leg cramps.

> *But LORD, be merciful to us, for we have waited for you. Be our strength each day and our salvation in times of trouble.*
> —ISAIAH 33:2

Low Blood Sugar

Many people develop low blood sugar during the night, and as a result they have restless sleep. When the blood sugar level drops, certain hormones are released by the body to raise the blood sugar as rapidly as possible. These hormones include adrenaline, cortisol and glycogen. As a result, the body is jolted awake by the brain telling the body that it's time to eat. By simply eating a bedtime snack of whole-grain bread, pasta, oatmeal, low-fat yogurt (or for overweight individuals I recommend a Balance bar), you will usually prevent low blood sugar during the night. These carbohydrates will help to raise the level of serotonin, which will keep you sleeping soundly.

If you have candida, you should avoid starches and yogurt, and eat a salad with olive oil and lemon juice instead.

Conclusion

The Bible Cure pathway to decreasing fatigue and increasing your strength and energy daily is to get enough sleep. It's time for you to rest in the Lord and let go of habits and overcome physical problems that interrupt your sleep.

God promises to give you rest and increase your strength. Your Bible Cure promise is found in the well-known Twenty-third Psalm. I have adapted that psalm as a Bible Cure prayer for you to pray daily as you seek His rest and strength.

A Bible Cure Prayer
FOR YOU

Lord, You are my shepherd; I have everything I need.

Thank You for letting me rest in green meadows and leading me beside peaceful streams.

I praise You for renewing my strength. Lord, guide me along right paths, that I might bring honor to Your name.

Even when I walk through the dark valley of death, I will not be afraid, for You are close beside me. Your rod and Your staff protect and comfort me.

You prepare a feast for me in the presence of my enemies. You welcome me as a guest, anointing my head with oil. My cup overflows with blessings.

Surely Your goodness and unfailing love will pursue me all the days of my life, and I will live in the house of the Lord forever. Amen.

—ADAPTED FROM PSALM 23

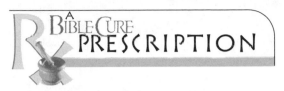

A BIBLE CURE PRESCRIPTION

In order to rest properly, you must eliminate certain things from your life. Check those things below that you will eliminate and avoid:

- ❏ Caffeine
- ❏ Sleeping pills
- ❏ Alcohol

Check the positive steps you will take:

- ❏ Get seven to eight hours of sleep regularly.
- ❏ If you have restless leg syndrome, consult with a physician about your possible need of iron, calcium or more testing for sleep disorders.

Write a prayer thanking God for His rest, care and peace in your life:

_____

_____

_____

Chapter 5

Restore With
Vitamins and Supplements

Your body is a masterful balance of artistry and chemistry, a perfect design of creative genius. God alone could create you—you were intricately and wonderfully made by Him! The Bible states, "You made all the delicate, inner parts of my body and knit me together in my mother's womb. Thank you for making me so wonderfully complex! Your workmanship is marvelous—and how well I know it. You watched me as I was being formed in utter seclusion, as I was woven together in the dark of the womb" (Ps. 139:13–15).

The divine Creator has also supplied countless sources of energy to restore, strengthen and nourish this wonderful machine. Vitamins and minerals are uniquely programmed by God to support the various systems of your body.

God desires for you to take care of your body, the temple of God's Spirit, so that you can live a fully abundant life serving Him. Although found in some measure in the foods we eat, taking supplemental vitamins and minerals will both strengthen your body and give you the vitality you need to overcome fatigue.

Don't be discouraged. Don't quit and don't give up. You will win out over fatigue! Trust His promise: "But those who wait on the LORD will find new strength. They will fly high on wings like eagles. They will run and not grow weary. They will walk and not faint" (Isa. 40:31).

> *The Sovereign LORD, the Holy One of Israel, says, "Only in returning to me and waiting for me will you be saved. In quietness and confidence is your strength."*
> —ISAIAH 30:15

Fight Back With Supplements

Vitamins and minerals are also important in the restoration of adrenal function. But do store shelves filled with bottles of vitamins leave you feeling a little mystified? Here is some basic, vital information about the supplements and vitamins that you can take to begin feeling better once more.

Vitamin B$_5$, which is pantothenic acid, is extremely important during periods of stress. It is used in the production of ATP, and its deficiency is commonly associated with fatigue and sleep disturbances. It will eventually result in atrophy of the adrenal glands. Vitamin B$_5$ is found in cruciferous vegetables such as broccoli and cauliflower. It is also found in whole grains, legumes, tomatoes and salmon.

I recommend a dose of approximately 250 milligrams, two times a day. For individuals with severe adrenal exhaustion, I recommend up to 500 milligrams, twice daily. I also recommend taking a B-complex vitamin that contains at least 50 milligrams of the B vitamins, two to three times a day.

Zinc is also important in restoring adrenal function. I recommend at least 30 milligrams a day. I also recommend at least 400 milligrams of magnesium daily.

Vitamin C is also necessary during periods of excessive stress or when you have developed adrenal exhaustion. During periods of excessive stress, your kidneys tend to flush extra vitamin C from your body. Therefore, supplement with at least 500 to 1,000 milligrams, two to three times a day in order to preserve immune function during these times.

5-HTP is one of many different natural supplements that will help to relieve insomnia and produce good quality sleep. 5-HTP, otherwise known as 5-hydroxytryptophan, is a form of tryptophan, which is an amino acid that is a step closer to forming the neurotransmitter serotonin. Serotonin is extremely important in both improving the quality of your sleep and helping you to fall asleep.

5-HTP actually improves the quality of sleep by increasing the time spent in REM sleep, and also by increasing the time spent in stages three and four of phase one, which are the deeper stages of sleep. The amount of time spent in superficial sleep, stages one and two, is actually decreased. However, these are the least important stages of sleep. The total time of sleep is not prolonged. In other words, you will spend more time in deeper sleep, have more time in REM sleep causing more dreaming and thus awaken more refreshed.

Like the example of recharging a golf cart, if you were able to improve both your sleep quality and the time spent in REM sleep, you would be able to fully charge your physical and mental batteries. This would provide more energy, mental clarity and possibly even more creativity during the day.

Normally, I recommend approximately 100 to 500 milligrams of 5-HTP thirty minutes to an hour prior to going to bed. Higher doses of 5-HTP can sometimes produce nightmares; therefore, start low and gradually increase the dosage until sleep quality has improved. It is best to take the 5-HTP with fruit or some applesauce unless you have candida.

A multivitamin. Take a comprehensive multivitamin that contains adequate amounts of magnesium, niacin and B$_6$, which are important cofactors in converting 5-HTP to serotonin.

Melatonin is a hormone secreted by the pineal gland. It is also important in both helping you fall asleep and maintaining your sleep. Melatonin, however, only produces a sedative or a sleep-inducing effect when the levels of melatonin in the body are low. This is usually the case in elderly patients. In younger patients, the melatonin levels are usually normal; therefore, melatonin is unlikely to produce sedative effects. I normally recommend a dose of 1 to 3 milligrams of melatonin at bedtime.

DSF. Finally, I recommend a supplement by Nutri-West called "DSF," which stands for *de-stress formula*. This supplement contains pantothenic acid, zinc, magnesium, niacinamide, B_6 and other vitamins and minerals, along with adrenal-glandular extract, and thymus, spleen, stomach and parotid glandular extracts. This supplement is very effective in helping to restore adrenal function, and I recommend it routinely in my practice.

DHEA. Another important substance that I often recommend, especially in men, is DHEA. Before placing a patient on DHEA, I always check the DHEA sulfate level and the PSA level, which is the prostate specific antigen level. I recheck the DHEA sulfate level approximately one to three months later. I recheck the PSA level approximately six months later.

DHEA is actually a precursor for almost all of the steroid hormones in the body, including sex hormones and cortisol. As we age, the level of DHEA declines. When those who were previously deficient in DHEA receive safe doses, they can experience strength and vigor they haven't had for years. It also helps to relieve chronic fatigue. The individual is thus able to manage stress better, and this, in turn, decreases the stress on the adrenal glands. This gives the adrenals a rest, increasing the opportunity to restore their function.

If you have chronic fatigue syndrome you

probably have a low immune function. In order to improve immune function you must take the stress off the adrenal glands, and you must improve the function of the thymus. Thymus glandular extracts are usually quite effective for this.

Again, I recommend the DSF formula, which has both adrenal and thymus extract in order to help support both the adrenal and thymus gland.

Antioxidants. In addition to glandular extracts, I recommend adequate amounts of antioxidants—vitamin E, vitamin C, beta carotene, selenium, zinc, grapeseed extract and so forth. Please refer to my book *Walking in Divine Health* (Creation House) for more information concerning antioxidants.

Herbs That Energize

Valerian is an herb that comes from the valerian root. This herb has been used for centuries to treat insomnia and nervous conditions. Valerian also contains certain essential oils that may contribute to its sedating properties. Valerian has the ability to increase the deeper stages of sleep (stages three and four). The usual dose of valerian root extract is 150 to 300 milligrams. However, many people take as much as 500 milligrams, approximately one hour before bedtime.

Passionflower is another herb that has been used for treating insomnia for over a hundred years. Flavonoids in this herb are considered responsible for its sedating and anti-anxiety properties. Passionflower is commonly combined with valerian, which enhances its sedating properties. The Aztec Indians used passionflower as a sedative centuries ago. Both passionflower and valerian can also be taken with 5-HTP at bedtime. The normal dosage of passionflower is approximately 300 to 450 milligrams.

Ginseng. Certain herbs are also very important in restoring adrenal function. The first one is ginseng. Siberian ginseng and Chinese ginseng are two of a number of different varieties of ginseng. Chinese ginseng, otherwise known as *Panax ginseng,* has been used for centuries as an adaptogen. An adaptogen is an innocuous substance that is able to normalize a wide variety of pathological states. Both Chinese and Siberian ginseng can enhance adrenal function, thus helping you to tolerate stressful events better. It enables the body to resist fatigue and stress, preventing adrenal exhaustion.

Taking ginseng often helps people to cope better under both mental and physical stress. Both

Chinese and Siberian ginseng also protect the adrenals by blocking the alarm phase of the stress reaction, which is the "fight or flight" response. Thus, a person is not left to "stew in his own juices" as adrenaline shoots through his body. Chinese ginseng is the stronger of the two. It helps individuals under extreme stress or those who have been on long-term cortisone treatments. For milder forms of stress, Siberian ginseng is usually very effective.

An effective dose of ginseng is usually 100 milligrams, twice a day. Many individuals can only tolerate it in the morning and early afternoon, and some people can only tolerate it in the morning, since it tends to energize the body. After taking this recommended dosage for approximately eight weeks, take a one to two week break.

> *I am praying to you because I know you will answer, O God. Bend down and listen as I pray. Show me your unfailing love in wonderful ways. You save with your strength those who seek refuge from their enemies. Guard me as the apple of your eye. Hide me in the shadow of your wings.*
> —PSALM 17:6–8

Licorice is a very effective in the treatment of chronic fatigue and helping to restore adrenal function. Licorice may also increase cortisol levels and prolong the half-life of cortisol. By doing this, the adrenals are able to rest and get restored. Licorice may be taken as a tincture, about ½ to 1 teaspoon, three times a day. It can also be taken in licorice root capsules, as much as 1 gram three times a day. If you experience problems with water retention and high blood pressure at this dosage level, you should be followed by a nutritional doctor, especially for blood pressure monitoring.

St. John's Wort. If your chronic fatigue includes the additional symptoms of fibromyalgia, St. John's Wort may help. This herb acts as an antidepressant. Take 300 milligrams three times a day.

A BIBLE CURE HEALTH TIP

Energize With Supplements

To help you increase your energy level, I've listed my own supplement program, which boosts my energy tremendously:

1. A comprehensive multivitamin formula. I take the Divine Health Multivitamin for Men. This contains

optimal amounts of B vitamins, water and fat-soluble vitamins, minerals and antioxidants.

2. NADH, 5 milligrams, two times a day

3. Coenzyme Q_{10}, 50 milligrams, two times a day

4. Divine Health Green Superfood, one scoop, twice a day, which contains high amounts of chlorophyll foods, including wheat grass, barley grass, alfalfa, spirulina, ginkgo biloba, chlorella, soy lecithin, bee pollen, Siberian ginseng, good bacteria and antioxidants (including grapeseed extract and green tea).

5. DSF formula, which contains nutritional support for the adrenal glands. I take one of these twice a day.

By following this basic nutritional program, obtaining adequate rest and avoiding sugar and most processed foods, I get the energy to run a busy medical practice and travel throughout the U.S. continually without becoming fatigued.

Supplements for Candidiasis

Listed below are supplements that will dramatically impact fatigue by eliminating candidiasis yeast. These herbs should be avoided by pregnant women.

1. **Olive leaf extract.** In the Bible the olive tree is called the tree of life. When Moses was on Mount Sinai, the holy anointing oil was made of olive oil, along with other herbs. (See Exodus 30:22–25.) Olive leaf extract actually kills fungi, yeast, viruses, bacteria and even parasites. I recommend olive leaf extract in a dose of 500 milligrams, two tablets, 3 to 4 times a day.

2. **Garlic** is another herb that is very effective in controlling *candida albacans.* Allicin is the active component in garlic that is responsible for its antifungal activity. Take 400 milligrams of garlic three times a day. Four hundred milligrams of garlic is equivalent to 4,000 micrograms of allicin potential.

3. **Citrus seed extract or grapefruit seed extract** is also very effective in controlling yeast. I recommend 200 milligrams three to four times a day.

4. **Pau d'arco or taheebo tea** comes from the Pau d'arco trees that are found in the rain forest in Latin America. Pau d'arco has potent antifungal properties. The normal dose is 300 milligrams, three capsules, three times a day.

5. **Berberines** are herbs that include barberry, goldenseal and Oregon graperoot. The different berberine herbs have potent antifungal properties as well as antibacterial properties. Therefore, they are able to control bacterial overgrowth in the small intestine as well as destroy yeast overgrowth in the small intestines.

   The normal dose of berberines is 500 milligrams of a standard berberine extract, three times a day. Many nutritional doctors will only use berberine extracts for three weeks and then take a break of at least two weeks. Berberine-containing plants, again, are not to be used during pregnancy.

6. **Caprylic acid** is a long chain fatty acid that is also present in coconuts. Caprylic acid is an effective treatment for yeast. The normal dose is 1000 to 2000 milligrams, three times a day with meals. It is best to take a time-released formula.

7. **Oil of oregano** should be enteric coated. It is also extremely effective against yeast and comes in tablet form. I recommend 50 milligrams of standardized oregano extract, three to five tablets, three times per day.

Medications

Nystatin is a medication used to treat yeast for over twenty years. It comes in both tablet and powder form. The tablet is 500,000 units per tablet, or ⅛ teaspoon of powder is equal to 500,000 units. I commonly place patients on nystatin in addition to the abovementioned herbal formulas. I start them on one tablet, or 500,000 units, three times a day and gradually increase them to a million units, three times a day.

I often use the powder. However, many patients dislike it. For patients who are able to tolerate the powder, I have them start with ⅛ teaspoon in 4 ounces of water, three times a day and gradually increase the dose to ¼ teaspoon, three to four times a day, again, with approximately 4 ounces of water. You may add fresh-squeezed lemon juice and Stevia to help conceal the taste.

> *It is useless for you to work so hard from early morning until late at night, anxiously working for food to eat; for God gives rest to his loved ones.*
> —PSALM 127:2

If the yeast persists, I prescribe Diflucan, Sporanox or Lamisil tablets. These three drugs have systemic antiyeast properties. Before starting these systemic antiyeast medications, I usually perform a comprehensive digestive stool analysis to determine what type of yeast a patient has and which medications or herbs the yeast responds to.

Conclusion

God has provided us with many supplements and

vitamins to restore health and energy to our lives. Through prayer and His Word you can be strengthened spiritually to make the best decisions for reducing chronic fatigue and discover the faith and strength you need to live life abundantly. As you defeat chronic fatigue and fibromyalgia, claim this Bible Cure promise for yourself and make it your prayer of praise:

> Praise the LORD, I tell myself; with my whole heart, I will praise his holy name. Praise the LORD, I tell myself, and never forget the good things he does for me. He forgives all my sins and heals all my diseases. He ransoms me from death and surrounds me with love and tender mercies. He fills my life with good things. My youth is renewed like the eagle's!
>
> —PSALM 103:1–5

A BIBLE CURE PRAYER
FOR YOU

Heavenly Father, I know that You alone can strengthen and guide me out of chronic fatigue and into Your strength and renewing power. I ask You for the wisdom to make right choices about reducing my stress, getting good nutrition, getting adequate sleep and taking the right vitamins and supplements for my body. Thank You for the temple of my body that I can care for and use for Your glory and service. Fill me now with strength. Give me peace and rest that I may be renewed daily to live abundantly in Your good plans for my life. Amen.

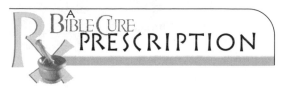

A BIBLE CURE PRESCRIPTION

List the vitamins you will take:

_____

List the supplements you need to be taking:

_____

List the herbs you will take:

_____

Complete these sentences:

The most important thing I learned about being energized with vitamins and supplements is

_____

_____ .

To overcome chronic fatigue, I daily need to

_____

_____ .

Chapter 6

Refresh With
the Power of Spiritual Joy

Have you felt overwhelmed by the dark weight of depression that often accompanies chronic fatigue and fibromyalgia? I have wonderful news for you. By faith you can hand that hopelessness and sadness to Jesus Christ, and in return He will refresh you with the power of spiritual joy!

If you are overwhelmed by fatigue, the cause may not be only physical. Your energy and vigor may be depleted by circumstances in your life that are taxing your energy and encumbering you. If so, turn immediately to God for strength and rest. Give your worries and cares to Him. (See 1 Peter 5:7.)

Worry and anxiety are ingredients of today's stressed-out lifestyle. Excessive stress may actually be the root cause of anxiety and depression. It weakens the immune system and may be a contributing factor in the development of cancer. Stress aggravates heart disease and even causes some heart attacks.

But God's plan for you does not include living under constant stress, worry and anxiety. Constant stress can produce depression and fatigue. God invites you to bring your worries and concerns to Him in prayer. In exchange for your anxieties, He will give you peace. "Don't worry about anything; instead, pray about everything. Tell God what you need, and thank him for all he has done. If you do this, you will experience God's peace, which is far more wonderful than the human mind can understand. His peace will guard your hearts and minds as you live in Christ Jesus" (Phil. 4:6–7).

> *The LORD is my strength and my song; he has become my victory. He is my God, and I will praise him; he is my father's God, and I will exalt him!*
> —Exodus 15:2

If you have been experiencing a great deal of sadness, you may be suffering from depression. Many chronic fatigue victims do. Following are some Bible Cure steps to take that will help.

Take the One-Year-to-Live Test

Suppose that you only have one year to live. What

would you choose to do and not do during that time? Group these activities into three different categories:

1. The things that you enjoy doing
2. The things that you must do
3. The things that you neither enjoy nor must do

You should eliminate all of the items in category number three. For the remainder of your life, try to forget about the activities that you neither enjoy nor have to do. Do not take on any projects or commitments that may be taxing to you for the next few months until your adrenal glands become strengthened.

Talk With a Counselor

If you are anxious, depressed, extremely angry or grieving over the loss of a loved one, then consider consulting professional help, such as the family doctor or a professional counselor. In order to work through and resolve these emotional conflicts, medication might be needed if the anxiety, depression or grief is severe. It is critically important to resolve these emotional conflicts in order to restore adrenal function.

Do you have unforgiveness hidden in your heart?

Many chronic fatigue and fibromyalgia sufferers do. Ask the Holy Spirit to reveal to you anyone you have not forgiven, and then release them.

Taking these steps together with the other Bible Cure principles outlined in this booklet will doubtless provide great relieve. But the most important Bible Cure step is not a physical one—it's spiritual.

Receive God's Wonderful Joy

The wonderful joy of God's refreshing presence washes away depression, sadness and fatigue. Jesus Christ came to trade your weariness and depression for His refreshing joy. He proclaimed His purpose in coming to ancient Israel through these words:

> The Spirit of the Sovereign Lord is on me, because the Lord has anointed me to preach good news to the poor. He has sent me to bind up the brokenhearted, to proclaim freedom to the captives and release from darkness for the prisoners . . . to comfort all who mourn, and provide for those who grieve in Zion—to bestow on them a crown of beauty instead of ashes, the oil of gladness instead of mourning, and a garment of praise instead of a spirit of despair.
>
> —Isaiah 61:1–3, NIV

That same Spirit did not leave the earth when Christ ascended after the resurrection. The anointing that comforts, refreshes, restores and renews is still here. His name is the Holy Spirit!

Jesus Christ loves you more than you'll ever know, and He paid a great price of death on a cross to heal, restore and refresh you. In addition, the precious Holy Spirit is right there with you, waiting for you to turn your eyes to Him. Why not bow

> *God is our refuge and strength, always ready to help in times of trouble. So we will not fear, even if earthquakes come and the mountains crumble into the sea.*
> —PSALM 46:1–2

your head and pray this simple prayer of faith and receive His gift of healing?

Faith Is So Simple

Let me share a wonderful truth with you about faith. Faith is not an eerie power or an extra-terrestrial force. Faith is a choice. It's a choice to believe God, no matter what your circumstances and feelings may be telling you. I've traveled around the world, and I've been blessed to witness hundreds of people rising up out of wheel-chairs, completely healed by God's wonderful presence (the very same presence that's with you chairs, completely healed by God's wonderful presence (the very same presence that's with you right now). These people weren't more spiritual than you are. They weren't more religious. They didn't come from generations of great preachers and saints. They were simply people who chose to believe God and believe what He said in His Book, the Bible. Faith is so simple!

Pray the Bible Cure prayer on this page, and then make the choice. Thank God for His wonderful promise and the incredible price He paid to give it to you. Then thank Him continually for His incredible love for you. I join my faith with yours, and I believe together with you that the strength and comfort of the Holy Spirit are yours right now!

A BIBLE CURE PRAYER
FOR YOU

Jesus, thank You for coming in the power of God's Holy Spirit to replace my sadness with joy and my sorrow with laughter. I receive the gift of Your healing power, Your restoration and Your salvation by faith. Thank You for Your great love for me and Your wonderful power to save me.

Conclusion

A New, Invigorated and Energized You!

The causes of chronic fatigue and fibromyalgia are complicated and numerous. But these diseases are not an end of vitality. I trust that as you take these Bible Cure steps, you will discover a new beginning. I encourage you to be committed to the many nutritional and lifestyle changes outlined in this little booklet. More importantly, keep your eyes on God as your source of healing, hope, restoration and renewal.

—DON COLBERT, M.D.

Notes

PREFACE
FRESH HOPE FOR A NEW YOU!

1. Leonard A. Jason, et. al., "A Community-Based Study of Chronic Fatigue Syndrome," *The Archives of Internal Medicine,* Vol. 959, No. 18, October 11, 1999, and information from CFIDS Asociation of America (www.cfids.org).

CHAPTER 1
KNOW YOUR ENEMY—UNDERSTANDING
CHRONIC FATIGUE AND FIBROMYALGIA

1. *The Archives of Internal Medicine,* Vol. 159, No. 18, October 11, 1999 and information from CFIDS Association of America (www.cfids.org).
2. Take a survey for yourself that is found on page 15 in *Yeast Connection* by Dr. William Crook (Professional Books/Future Health, Inc., reissued 1999).

CHAPTER 2
REFUEL WITH NUTRITION

1. Bill Krasean, *Antibiotics in Livestock a Human Risk* (8/11/98 Michigan Live, Inc.) www.kz.mlive.com.

Don Colbert, M.D., was born in Tupelo, Mississippi. He attended Oral Roberts School of Medicine in Tulsa, Oklahoma, where he received a bachelor of science degree in biology in addition to his degree in medicine. Dr. Colbert completed his internship and residency with Florida Hospital in Orlando, Florida. He is board certified in family practice and has received extensive training in nutritional medicine.

If you would like more
information about natural and
divine healing, or information about
Divine Health Nutritional Products®,
you may contact
Dr. Colbert at:

Dr. Don Colbert

1908 Boothe Circle
Longwood, FL 32750
Telephone: 407-331-7007

Dr. Colbert's website is
www.drcolbert.com.